College of Occupational Therapists' Learning and development standards for pre-registration education

Accreditation process

College of
Occupational
Therapists

First published in 2014
by the College of Occupational Therapists Ltd
106–114 Borough High Street
London SE1 1LB
www.cot.org.uk

Author: College of Occupational Therapists
Category: Education and development

Other enquiries about this document should be addressed to the Education and Learning Department at the above address.

British library Cataloguing in Publication Data
A catalogue record for this book is available from the British Library.

ISBN 978-1-905944-45-3

Typeset by Servis Filmsetting Ltd, Stockport, Cheshire
Digitally printed on demand in Great Britain by The Lavenham Press, Suffolk

FSC www.fsc.org
MIX
Paper from responsible sources
FSC® C010693

Contents

Throughout this document, 'a programme' and 'programmes' refer to pre-registration programmes only; the 'College' and 'COT' refer to the College of Occupational Therapists; 'HEI(s)' refer to higher education institution(s).

1 Introduction

The accreditation scheme offered by the College of Occupational Therapists ensures that occupational therapy pre-registration programmes in the United Kingdom (UK) meet the education standards and curriculum requirements set by the College as the only occupational therapy professional body in the UK.

The College of Occupational Therapists is the national body that defines the values, beliefs and philosophy of the occupational therapy profession and specifies the criteria for 'fitness for the occupational therapy profession' in the form of an entry-level profile for application to the regulatory register. It is the education, practice development and research arm of the British Association of Occupational Therapists (BAOT), the professional membership organisation that promotes excellence in the standards of delivery of occupational therapy practice and development in the UK.

The United Kingdom, through the BAOT, is a member country of the World Federation of Occupational Therapists (WFOT), the international voice for occupational therapists and occupational therapy around the world and the official international organisation for the promotion of occupational therapy. WFOT is a non-governmental organisation (NGO) recognised by the United Nations and has official standing with the World Health Organization. WFOT sets the global minimum standards for the education and training of occupational therapists and influences the development of excellence within the profession.

COT holds the delegated authority of the WFOT and therefore COT accreditation of a pre-registration programme confers both WFOT and COT recognition of the education provider and approval of the programme (www.wfot.org). This ensures that graduates of an accredited institution will hold a degree that is recognised by any country in the world belonging to the Federation.

The College sets the education standards for the accreditation of pre-registration programmes. Education providers that offer College accredited occupational therapy programmes are assured, therefore, that their programmes and graduates using the title 'occupational therapy' and 'occupational therapist':

- Are fit for academic award, practice, purpose and profession.
- Adhere to the latest curriculum framework of the COT.
- Meet the minimum standards for the education of occupational therapists set by the WFOT.
- Are responsive to local, national and global issues that influence the learning requirements of students of the profession.
- Are able to demonstrate that the College's professional standards for lifelong learning and the code of ethics and professional conduct are embedded within their programme.

The Health and Care Professions Council (HCPC) is the regulatory body for the allied health professions (AHPs) in the UK. It has been established by the government to protect the public. The HCPC maintains a register of health and care professionals who meet the HCPC standards for their training, professional skills, behaviour and health.

Mutual recognition and respect for each other's specific remit, that is, 'fitness for practice' for the HCPC and 'fitness for the profession' for the College of Occupational Therapists, are fundamental to the good working relationship between the College and the HCPC. This is particularly evident in the planning and conducting of tripartite approval events that involve the College, the HCPC and the HEI. The objectivity and professionalism of the College's accreditors and HCPC visitors are vital to maintaining this relationship. The education officers of the respective bodies work hard to maintain effective working relationships and good communication channels, from the planning of the event to the final outcome.

HCPC approval of a programme is a requirement for COT accreditation in view of the College's remit to ensure that a person successfully completing an accredited pre-registration programme is 'fit for the profession' and therefore fit for practice.

1.1 Document purpose

This document is intended to provide an overview of COT accreditation services, and:

- To introduce potential occupational therapy education providers to the role of the COT in pre-registration occupational therapy education in the UK and to describe the details and expectations of the COT accreditation cycle.
- To provide a clear guide to education providers seeking re-accreditation with the COT to describe the details and expectations of the COT accreditation process.
- To provide stakeholders involved in pre-registration education of occupational therapy students with an insight into the COT accreditation process, expectations and requirements.
- To demonstrate the rigour and ongoing commitment in achieving COT accredited status.

1.2 Benefits

- Assurance of automatic national and international recognition of the programme that should enhance student recruitment.
- Inclusion in the *Occupational therapy careers handbook* published annually by the COT on the website and distributed to careers advisers in the UK and potential students (viewed online nearly 100,000 times a year).
- Opportunity to highlight the benefits of COT recognition in student recruitment marketing materials for the programme (including permission to use the COT accreditation logo).
- Access to unparalleled professional expertise, experience and advice on occupational therapy pre-registration education.
- Access to support and advice to help address local issues in education provider institutions that are challenging to resolve or need additional professional expertise or support provided by the professional body.
- Opportunity to list all appropriate continuing professional development offerings on the COT website, viewed an average of 1000 times per day.

- Access to advice and information on leading-edge pre-registration and post-qualification education issues through position statements and guidance documents, including education policy briefings designed to guide the curriculum and enhance professional knowledge. Briefings are developed in collaboration with experienced educators, practitioners and other stakeholders.
- More opportunities to become part of established networks of occupational therapy education providers in the UK and internationally, through which intelligence, advice and knowledge are shared and strategic actions are developed and debated to ensure currency of programmes.
- Increased opportunities to participate in collaborative work with the College at a national level on issues relating to occupational therapy education provision and through the professional body's influencing activities at a strategic level.
- Access to up-to-date knowledge on government legislation and other publications by virtue of the unique position of the College, its education experts and reference groups to receive, search and sift this information.
- Increased opportunity to debate and respond to the potential impact of new issues relevant to occupational therapy learning and development.
- Access to collaborative work undertaken by the College with other health and allied health professional bodies (e.g. Allied Health Professions Forum, Royal College of Psychiatrists, Chartered Society of Physiotherapy, Royal College of Speech and Language Therapists), specialist organisations and government agencies (e.g. National Institute for Health and Clinical Effectiveness (NICE)).
- International recognition of programmes by the WFOT. Graduates will hold a degree that is recognised by any country belonging to that federation (subject to the requirements of the individual country's regulating body).
- Opportunity to work in partnership with COT in the development of the professional base to influence the evolution of progressive, cutting-edge occupational therapy, both nationally and internationally.
- Access to COT annual reports and data on student and graduate profiles, which are used to compare the HEI's own data against the national picture.
- Employers can be assured of:
  - graduates having successfully completed a programme that has passed the professional body's quality assurance of the core components of both theoretical studies and professional practice for safe practice of the profession;
  - the education provider having involved stakeholders and service users in the development and delivery of their programme.

1.3 Impact of non-accreditation

For the education provider:

- Programmes and education providers will not be granted approval by the WFOT. The occupational therapy qualification of graduates from non-accredited programmes will not be recognised in WFOT member countries. Prospective students may therefore choose not to enrol in these programmes.
- Non-accredited status of programmes will be highlighted in the *Occupational therapy careers handbook*, published annually by the College of Occupational Therapists and

distributed to careers advisers in the UK and potential students. Recruitment to these programmes may therefore be affected.

- No access to the regularly updated Register of External Examiners, which includes the entries of experienced educators in the UK who are eligible to be appointed as external examiners.
- No access to professional advice on curriculum development and current leading-edge pre-registration and post-qualification education and practice issues that may enhance programme quality and professional staff development.
- No access to professional advice on the management of student progression issues.
- Staff from non-accredited programmes would not be eligible to be a COT accreditor.

For the student:

- Graduates will not have completed a programme that has passed the professional body's quality assurance of the core components of both theoretical studies and professional practice for safe practice of the profession.
- Graduates will not have completed a programme that is recognised by the WFOT and therefore not be eligible to practise in member countries.
- Graduates cannot be assured that they have completed a programme in which employers, service users or carers have any confidence.

For the employer:

- A knowledge that graduates will not have completed a programme that has passed the professional body's quality assurance of the core components of both theoretical studies and professional practice for safe practice of the profession.
- Non-accredited programmes will not be included in COT annual reports on student and graduate profiles, which could be used to inform national workforce planning and occupational therapy education commissioning.

2 Accreditation and re-accreditation of pre-registration occupational therapy programmes

2.1 The role of accreditation

The purpose of accreditation is to ensure that:

- Graduates from accredited programmes are fit for the occupational therapy profession at a level beyond the 'fitness to practice' benchmark required for registration with the HCPC.
- Graduates from accredited programmes meet TUNING and WFOT standards.
- Graduates from accredited occupational therapy programmes are educated and practise in a manner that is consistent with the values, beliefs and philosophy of the profession, and by so doing demonstrate 'fitness for profession'.
- Education providers who work in partnership with the College will have confidence that their programmes accord with the highest possible standards for occupational therapy education and are forward thinking to future practice.

COT accreditation is not intended to award academic credits but to act as an enhanced quality benchmark for potential applicants, employers and commissioners when considering the merits and effectiveness of a particular programme in meeting the College's entry-level criteria.

2.2 Accreditation process

The College believes that occupational therapy programme accreditation and review/ re-accreditation are collaborative processes focused on quality assurance between the College and the HEI. It is not considered to be in the best interests of either party for a programme to fail to achieve COT accreditation. Thus, the College will do its best to advise the programme team on how COT criteria and standards can be achieved and thereby facilitate the process, where possible. Programme teams should seek help and support when developing and preparing the documentation for the accreditation process. Once documentation is submitted, the formal accreditation process is commenced and from this point the College will be acting as auditors of the programme and not as a critical friend.

Accreditation and re-accreditation will involve a visit by COT to the programme. This can be a joint event with the HEI and the HCPC. The visit requires discussion of the documentation with the programme team and senior management on site, as well as meetings with practice educators (with a visit to a placement setting, if requested) and students, and an inspection visit to the facilities and learning resources. See Figure 1 for the outline of the accreditation process and Figure 2 for re-accreditation below.

The COT Education Manager (Quality and Standards) is the first point of contact for information and advice on all aspects of the COT accreditation process and quality monitoring of programmes.

2.2.1 The timetable for accreditation

Review and re-accreditation will normally take place every five years, unless COT considers it necessary to revisit the programme earlier, for example:

- A programme with an inexperienced teaching team.
- A rapid turnover of staff since the last accreditation event.
- Where major changes are being introduced to the curriculum.
- If the submitted programme is highly innovative in its content, delivery and/or assessment.

An education provider may request an early or delayed review or re-accreditation in writing to COT for consideration. This application should include the rationale for the request.

The College would normally schedule an event to take place not later than June for a programme starting the following September and not later than October for a programme starting the following January.

Education providers are strongly advised to contact the COT preferably 12 months prior to the proposed start date of the programme, or earlier, for example as soon as they are successful in their bid for funding of the programme.

It would be advisable to offer a few possible dates for the event so that these can be entered in the accreditation events diary and ensure the availability of the most appropriate accreditors. The Education Manager (Quality and Standards) will also be able to advise immediately whether or not the dates proposed are acceptable or make alternative suggestions.

While it would be preferable and practicable to have a joint event with the HCPC, the HEI may choose to hold separate events for the regulatory body and the COT. The timetable and contents are generally similar to those suggested by the HCPC for both events.

2.2.2 Preparation for accreditation/re-accreditation visit

The College requires the submission of the documentation at least six weeks prior to the accreditation/re-accreditation event. The documentation may be requested in hard or soft copy by the College's accreditors. The College acknowledges that there is common information required by the university, the HCPC and the College to be included in the submission document, therefore the College would not expect the university to produce a separate document for COT accreditation that is different from that submitted to the university and the HCPC. However, COT would expect to find incorporated within the relevant sections of the submission document any additional information and specific professional regulations required by the College. These curriculum requirements and education standards are detailed in the College of Occupational Therapists' (2014) *Learning and development standards for pre-registration education*. The programme team is advised to cross-reference these requirements and standards against their submission document.

For re-accreditation, in addition to the submission document and any other documentation submitted to the HCPC, the following information should be included:

- Full programme appraisal from the most recent accreditation.
- External examiners' reports for the last two years.
- Rationale for changes to the curriculum.

Figure 1: Accreditation process flowchart

HEI is successful in obtaining funding for provision of an occupational therapy pre-registration programme.

↓

HEI informs COT of intention to submit a pre-registration occupational therapy programme for accreditation.

↓

COT Education Officer sends out information on COT accreditation to HEI.

↓

HEI pays accreditation fee.

↓

For a new programme (where no pre-registration occupational therapy programme is currently being delivered) the HEI should appoint the programme director/professional lead a minimum of 12 months prior to the start of the occupational therapy (OT) programme.

For a new additional programme (joining an established professional suite), the HEI should appoint the programme lead a minimum of six months prior to the start of the OT programme.

Advice from COT is available on request with regard to assisting with the appointment.

↓

Programme director writes the programme submission document

HEI to propose possible dates for accreditation event (these may be the same dates proposed to the HCPC).

↓

Date of the accreditation and approval event identified

COT Education Officer sends draft event timetable to HEI and informs HEI of names and contact details of COT accreditors (HEI will be invited to comment if aware of any conflict of interest).

↓

Six weeks prior to the accreditation event

HEI sends full set of submission documents to the COT panel together with the proposed agenda (taking account of HEI, COT and HCPC requirements).

↓

Accreditation event

↓

HEI advised of event outcome

Accreditation without conditions and/or recommendations

Accreditation with conditions and/or recommendations (date set for completion)

Deferred accreditation (resubmission within agreed timeframe)

↓

Where appropriate HEI submits evidence that they have met conditions and/or recommendations for consideration by COT within agreed timeframe.

↓

COT accreditation panel recommends approval to the College's Head of Education and Learning once satisfied that conditions and recommendations are met.

↓

Head of Education and Learning (COT) considers outcome of event (and additional evidence as appropriate) and confers accreditation status on the HEI.

↓

HEI details included in COT careers handbook and website. COT notifies WFOT.

↓

Ongoing accreditation arrangements put in place.

Figure 2: Re-accreditation process flowchart

HEI informs COT of its intention of submitting a pre-registration occupational therapy programme for re-accreditation

↓

Programme Director writes the submission document

HEI to propose possible dates for re-accreditation event proposed (these may be the same dates proposed to the HCPC).

↓

Date of the re-accreditation and approval event identified

COT Education Officer sends draft event timetable to HEI and informs HEI of names and contact details of COT accreditors (HEI will be invited to comment if aware of any conflict of interest).

↓

Six weeks prior to the re-accreditation event

HEI sends full set of submission documents sent to COT accreditors together with the proposed agenda (taking account of HEI, COT and HCPC requirements).

↓

Re-accreditation event

↓

HEI advised of event outcome

Re-accreditation without conditions and/or recommendations

Re-accreditation with conditions and/or recommendations (date set for completion)

Deferred re-accreditation (resubmission within agreed timeframe)

↓

Where appropriate HEI submits evidence that it has met conditions and/or recommendations for consideration by COT within agreed timeframe.

↓

COT accreditation panel recommends approval to the College's Head of Education and Learning once satisfied that conditions and recommendations are met.

↓

Head of Education and Learning (COT) considers outcome of event (and additional evidence as appropriate) and confers re-accreditation status on the HEI.

↓

HEI details included in COT careers handbook and website. COT notifies WFOT.

↓

Ongoing accreditation arrangements put in place.

2.2.3 COT requirements for the visit

COT has the following requirements for the accreditation visit:

- A discussion of the documentation with the programme team – this should be timetabled within the first half of the accreditation visit (where the visit's duration is more than one day, this meeting should take place on the first day) and can include a short, succinct presentation.
- A discussion with senior managers from the school/faculty and university (including the finance manager where appropriate) for the purpose of discussing resources, life span, commitment, staffing strategy.
- Meetings with practice educators and students (from all years and programmes).
- An inspection visit of the facilities and learning resources.

- COT may also request a visit to a placement site if deemed appropriate by the COT panel.

2.2.4 Accreditation/re-accreditation visit

Accreditation and re-accreditation will involve a visit by the COT accreditation panel to the HEI and programme team. This can be a joint event with the HEI and the HCPC. The COT accreditation panel members attending the visit will normally be comprised of the COT officer and a COT accreditor.

The COT officer is a member of the College staff and has the following roles throughout the accreditation process:

- To liaise with the host HEI Quality Office regarding the remit and expectations of the COT panel.
- To guide the COT panel members through the various panel and private meetings.
- To provide guidance on points of professional body regulation.
- To ensure that the COT panel addresses the requirements and standards of the College of Occupational Therapists' (2014) *Learning and development standards for pre-registration education.*
- To ensure that relevant conditions, recommendations and commendations are presented where required or a statement regarding the procedure following the visit is provided.
- To ensure that timely responses from the programme team following an event are dealt with.
- To manage the process internal to COT to the point of final outcome by the Head of Education and Learning.
- To liaise with the HEI Quality Office and programme team following the final outcome from the Head of Education and Learning.

The COT accreditor is a registered occupational therapist and member of the BAOT in good standing. Accreditors will have a range of experience in occupational therapy pre-registration education and practice. Those who are occupational therapy educators will be from COT accredited programmes. COT accreditors also assist the College in the quality monitoring of COT accredited programmes. See Section 3 for further details.

Two COT accreditors will be appointed to the COT accreditation panel. Both will act as reviewers of the submission documentation and will undertake discussions to inform the COT panel's initial discussion agenda. Only one accreditor will attend the visit with the COT officer. Both accreditors will be involved in the development of the outcome of the visit and review of any conditions and/or recommendations.

It should be noted that if the higher education provider appoints a critical friend/external expert to work with the programme team in the programme's development and through its validation process, this person may not then act as a COT accreditor.

Where a new occupational therapy pre-registration programme is being established or where two or more pre-registration programmes are being considered at the same event, the COT accreditation panel will consist of two COT accreditors and the COT officer.

2.2.5 Agenda for accreditation event

Please note that the final agenda will be by mutual agreement of participating stakeholders.

Example 1: COT model agenda for an accreditation event (new programme)

Agenda for accreditation event

(Chaired by HEI)

Day 1 agenda to include the following:

- Meeting with full panel to share identified issues to raise with the Programme Development Team (PDT) – venues/times to be decide by university.
- Initial meeting with PDT and Teaching Team.

Day 2 agenda to include the following:

- Agenda setting with the full panel.
- Inspection tour of accommodation, resources and facilities.
- Meeting with university senior management (Dean of Faculty, Head of School) to explore resource issues.
- Meeting with PDT to discuss further issues on the curriculum, practice education and programme regulations.
- Meeting with potential practice educators.

Where more than one occupation therapy pre-registration programme is being considered at the same event:

- Private meeting for the COT panel.
- COT may give initial feedback (as appropriate) to the event.

Example 2: COT model agenda for a re-accreditation event

Agenda for accreditation event

(Chaired by HEI)

Day 1 agenda to include the following:

- AM: COT accreditors visit practice placements, if required (accompanied by staff).
- Meeting with full panel to share identified issues to raise with the PDT – venues/times to be decide by university.
- Initial meeting with PDT and Teaching Team.

Day 2 agenda to include the following:

- Agenda setting with the full panel.

- Inspection tour of accommodation, resources and facilities.
- Meeting with students from across all years and all programmes.
- Meeting with practice educators.
- Meeting with the University Senior Management (Dean of Faculty, Head of School and Finance Managers and Commissioners as appropriate) to explore resource issues.
- Meeting with PDT to discuss further issues on the curriculum, practice education and programme regulations.

Where more than one occupation therapy pre-registration programme is being considered at the same event:

- Private meeting for the COT panel.
- COT may give initial feedback (as appropriate) to the event.

2.2.6 Outcome from accreditation/re-accreditation visit

The COT accreditation panel at the conclusion of the accreditation visit will usually provide verbal feedback to the programme (development) team. This feedback will give a flavour of conditions/recommendations that COT may require from the programme. The COT accreditation panel may also take the opportunity to make commendations. The final wording of the outcome from the College's panel will be sent to the higher education provider within one week of the visit.

The outcome may be:

- Accreditation with no conditions and/or recommendations.
- Accreditation subject to conditions and/or recommendations.
- Deferred accreditation (resubmission required and date agreed).

Where accreditation is granted with conditions and/or recommendations, the College's panel will agree with the programme team a date by which the conditions must be met. The programme team may consult the College's panel for advice on how the COT conditions and recommendations may be achieved.

An accreditation decision may be deferred when the College panel requires further information or evidence that the programme as a whole will meet the College of Occupational Therapists' (2014) *Learning and development standards for pre-registration education*. A mutually agreed timeframe will be set by the COT panel and the HEI in which responses and documentation will be sent to panel members for further consideration. A further meeting may also be required to discuss the additional documentation in order to reach a positive accreditation outcome.

A *condition* is defined as an obligation that must be met before the programme can be accredited. A condition is set where an education standard or curriculum requirement of the College has not been met or there is insufficient evidence of an education standard or curriculum requirement of the College being met.

A *recommendation* is defined as professional or academic advice that is intended to stimulate debate in order to encourage further enhancements to a programme. The provider is obligated to respond to the recommendation and to justify its response; however, it is not obliged to concur with the advice. Recommendations are normally offered when it is felt that the particular standard or curriculum requirement has been met at or just above the threshold level.

Commendations are awarded to recognise a particular area of best practice that is considered exemplary against peers at the time of award. It should be noted that a commendation is not a global statement across the programme, but rather is specific to the area of practice being recognised.

When conditions and recommendations have been met, the final recommendation for accreditation will be submitted by the College's panel to the College's Head of Education and Learning for approval. Once approval has been granted, the COT officer will send formal confirmation to the higher education provider. The College's accreditation activity will be reported to the College's Learning and Development Board and WFOT formally on an annual basis.

2.2.7 Evaluation/feedback of accreditation/re-accreditation visit

COT will undertake a system of feedback and review. Programme leads, the COT officer and COT accreditors will be asked to review each event. Any specific concerns raised by the programme lead in his or her feedback will be investigated by the Head of Education and Learning and formal feedback provided. The review information will be used to monitor, evaluate and quality assure the College's accreditation process and to inform the annual accreditation report to the College's Learning and Development Board.

2.2.8 Logo and its use

Once accreditation status is awarded by COT, an accreditation logo will be forwarded to the programme lead. Conditions of its use will accompany it. Failure to adhere to these conditions may lead to COT removing accreditation status for the programme.

2.3 Common preparation errors

Examples of common errors when preparing for the accreditation process:

- The appointment of practitioners with little or no background or experience in higher education to the post of programme director/professional programme lead. This has resulted in the development of a programme with no coherent occupational therapy education philosophy and a curriculum with a limited range of occupational therapy tools presented to students.
- A narrow or specialist approach to the design of the programme as articulated in its education and/or occupational therapy philosophy that would disadvantage a student's learning experience.
- Assessments failing to match the learning outcomes for each level.
- Absence of or failure to demonstrate in the document the process for monitoring and investigating a student's professional suitability and unsuitability.
- Regulations that do not conform to the College of Occupational Therapists' standards and curriculum requirements.
- Lack of clarity of resources.

- Failure to demonstrate in the documentation how the COT standards for education are met (cross-referencing).
- Failure to observe the College's position statement on lifelong learning in relation to professional staff's active engagement with professional and educational development through a range of activities, including scholarship and research.

2.4 Retrospective programme accreditation

The College does not grant retrospective accreditation of pre-registration programmes. This accords with the requirements of the WFOT.

Application for accreditation by a programme already running or a programme whose accreditation has previously expired can be made. However, only new students entering in the academic year following accreditation being awarded can be classified as having completed a WFOT approved programme.

In the case of currently accredited programmes seeking continued accreditation, the HEI has the option to apply for an extension to the programme's accreditation period.

Examples of legitimate reasons for extension requests include:

- Bringing an occupational therapy programme accreditation cycle in line with other AHP programmes in the HEI.
- Reorganisation of facilities/schools in an HEI.

Examples of non-legitimate reasons for extension requests include:

- Staff holidays.

Any request for an extension to the programme's period of accreditation must be made in writing, at least six months prior to the end date of the programme, to the Education Manager (Quality and Standards).

2.5 Ongoing quality monitoring

The COT accreditation scheme has an ongoing quality assurance process. This process requires the HEI to meet the continued requirements of the College listed in 2.5.1.

2.5.1 Requirements for continued COT accreditation

By receiving accreditation status a higher education provider agrees to:

- Adhere to the most recent education standards and curriculum requirements or any amendments consequently of the COT.
- Complete an annual report on each programme of study (to the deadline given) using the template provided, which is based on a self-declaration by the HEI as to their ability to continue to meet the education standards and curriculum requirements (COT 2014).
- Provide student lists annually (cohort and pass lists) and notification of student permanent or temporary withdrawal from their programme.

- Provide copies annually of the external examiner reports and the response made by the programme team/HEI to those reports.
- Advise COT of any major or minor change prior to the time of the change.
- Work proactively and in partnership with the College throughout the period of accreditation.
- Meet all the conditions required at the point of accreditation and undertake to report on the successful meeting of any conditions required at a later date (which were made as a condition of accreditation).

Failure to meet the requirements of the College may lead to the withdrawal of accreditation status from the higher education provider.

Copies of the annual report template are available on the College's website (www.cot.org.uk) or from the COT Education Manager (Quality and Standards). Normally, a request for completion of the report will be sent out at the end of the academic year, with a clear deadline for completion and return. It is expected that external examiner reports and the programme team's/HEI's response will also be attached to this return.

2.6 Process for approval of minor and major change

When a higher education provider makes a change to the accredited programme, COT must be informed prior to the change being implemented. The College requires written notification of the changes being made and the rationale, as well as the process for consideration of the changes that are being undertaken internally and whether HCPC or other stakeholders are involved.

On receipt of the planned change, COT will consider any impact to accreditation of the programme and will notify the higher education provider of any further information required. The provider will be advised of the expected timeframe for the outcome of the College's consideration. It is recommended that the provider allows a minimum of four months for the approval process; applications submitted with a shorter lead time may not be able to be considered and approved in time for the planned programme implementation date, creating a potential gap in COT accreditation.

All changes made will be recorded by the College and where the accrued record of changes is deemed to substantially alter the accredited programme, COT reserves the right to request further discussion with the higher education provider to ensure that the totality continues to meet COT's education standards and curriculum requirements.

The decision on the process of consideration to be observed shall lie with the College and may involve the review of material by a COT accreditor and discussion with the programme team.

Approval of a major or minor change does not alter the accreditation timeframe. All programmes will continue to be reviewed on their established five-year cycle regardless of whether a change has been approved within the programme's five-year accreditation cycle.

2.7 COT process for raising a concern with a university

A cause for concern may be raised by the College if:

- It is believed that the accredited HEI is not meeting the requirements of accreditation.
- The College receives a concern about the HEI or programme (raised by a student occupational therapist or a member of the public or profession).
- A potential issue is identified through the annual quality assurance process.

On receipt of a cause for concern about a programme, the process shown in Figure 3 will be enacted.

Figure 3: Management of a cause for concern

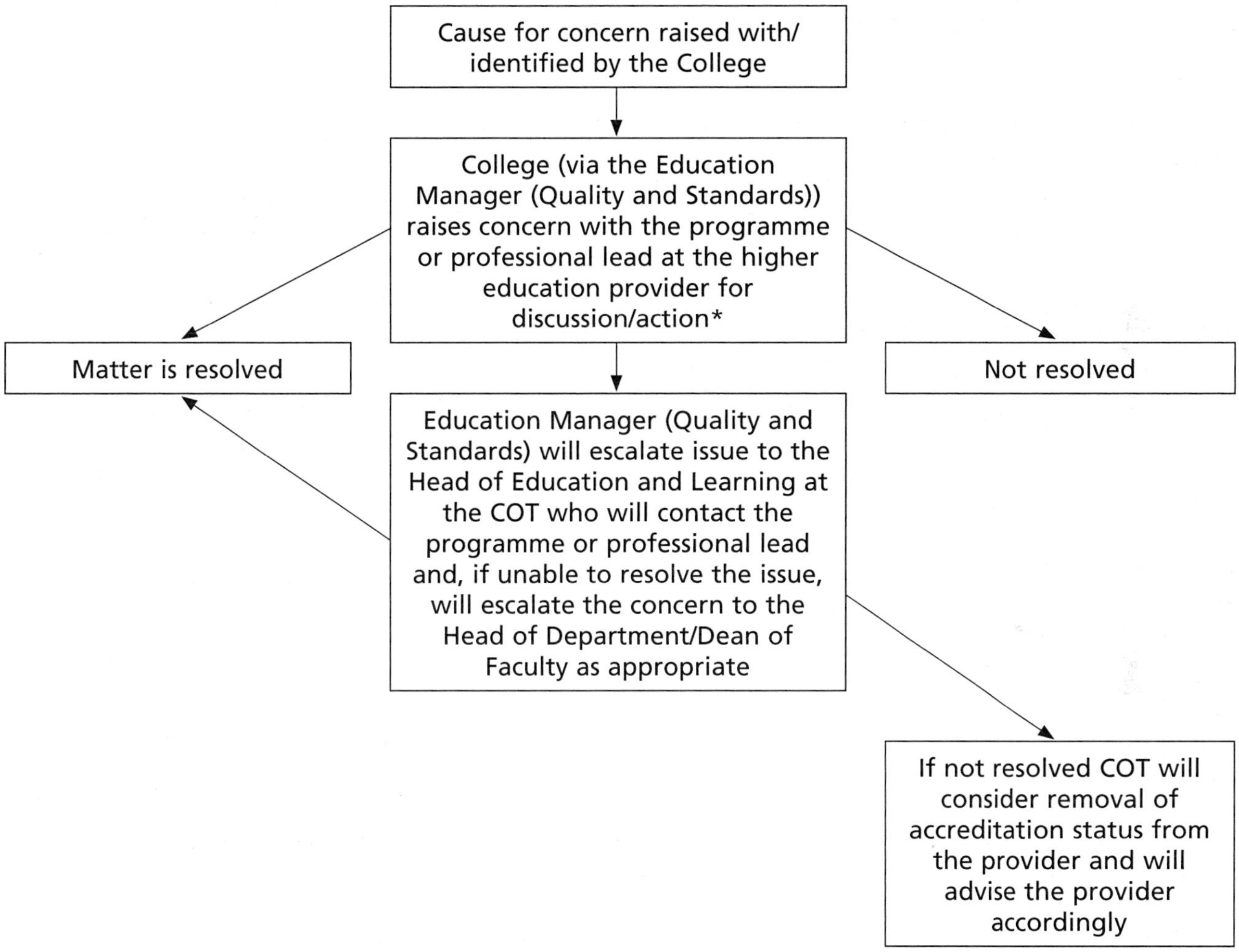

NB * The College may communicate with the HCPC depending on the nature of the concern.

In the event of the higher education provider wanting to raise a concern against the COT's accreditation services, these should be directed to the Head of Education and Learning in the first instance.

2.8 Requesting extensions for student studies

The College within its 2014 *Learning and development standards for pre-registration education* sets out the maximum time in which students will normally complete their studies. This is to ensure that those qualifying have currency of professional knowledge for safe practice and protection of the public.

Extension of a student's registration of no more than six months beyond the maximum time set by the COT may be requested, which must have prior approval of the College and have the support of the HEI. Requests for student extensions must be made by the HEI, in writing, addressed to the Education Manager (Quality and Standards). The request should include details of:

- The reason the request is being made and details of the circumstances leading to it.
- Confirmation of the student's journey to date (including commencement date and levels and stages completed within it).
- The student's academic profile.
- Details of any fitness to practise panel hearings.
- A statement as to whether the programme team is supportive of the request.
- Confirmation that funding arrangements have been discussed and agreed with the student.
- A plan detailing how the student would be supported through this additional period of study.

2.9 Charges and services associated with accreditation services

An accreditation charge is made to each HEI that delivers occupational therapy pre-registration programme(s). This fee includes a range of services (Figure 4).

Figure 4

The accreditation charge includes the following services
Professional body accreditation, continuing approval and periodic re-approval of all pre-registration education programmes, which includes: • Recognition by the professional body as an approved provider of education programmes; • External quality assurance that the education provision in individual institutions is at the appropriate standard, using robust peer-review processes aligned to institution's own procedures.
Access to external examiners register (Further advice and guidance is also provided by COT in relation to the individual HEIs' needs.)
Advice, guidance and support according to individual education providers' needs (e.g. advice on innovation and development in curriculum design and content; learning, teaching and assessment methods, etc.). Where COT staff are not available, details of experienced educators will be provided with their consent.
For newly appointed programme leads, COT will provide advice and guidance on suitable experienced educators who may act as mentors and will make available contact details with their consent.
Advice, guidance and support to individual education providers' needs on lobbying for student commissions, workforce development etc.
Local mediation services Where COT staff are not available, details of experienced educators will be provided with their consent.
Opportunity for programme team staff to be considered for attendance at COT-led study days (e.g. new external examiners, accreditors).

Periodic analytical reports on education that enable institutions to review their own provision against the overall UK picture. (This includes copies of annual reports supplying national data on student profiles, education provision, and related academic matters. Individual reports on the institutions' BAOT student membership data available on request.)
Travel, subsistence and, where appropriate, speakers' fees for professional body officers and staff asked to present at, or participate in, HEI events such as research conferences, graduation events, study days etc. (not including recruitment or induction to the profession) (normally to a maximum of one visit per HEI per year)
Provision of induction to the profession or BAOT recruitment sessions for current students (normally to a maximum of two visits per HEI per year).
Provision of professional body policy and guidance documents. Copies of core professional body publications sent directly to HEI subject librarians.
Opportunity to advertise short courses, continuing professional development opportunities etc. on relevant section of the COT website (to a maximum of ten per annum).
Formal qualifications (such as foundation degrees, HNCs, postgraduate diplomas, MScs) endorsed by the College.
National recruitment initiatives and activity that encourages prospective students to apply for education programmes.
Inclusion in the annual careers handbook and careers enquiry service. (All accredited HEIs are listed in the printed version of the handbook. Full programme details are available on the COT website and to careers enquirers.)
Advice and support to education providers and students on registering and activating BAOT student membership.
Inclusion of the education provider in the APPLE and APPLE (Support) schemes. Access and editing rights to the relevant section of the APPLE database, its contents and report functions for one named contact.

When the College is informed that a higher education provider wishes to develop a new occupational therapy pre-registration programme and seek accreditation, an invoice will be raised for the accreditation charge.

Where a programme is accredited but is not recruited to, COT accreditation will remain in place for two academic years. If the course is recruited to and runs after that time, COT will seek a formal re-accreditation discussion event to ensure that the programme remains fit for profession.

A current fee schedule is available by contacting education@cot.co.uk

3 COT accreditors

A COT accreditor is a registered occupational therapist and member of the BAOT in good standing. Accreditors will have a range of experience in occupational therapy pre-registration education and practice. Those who are occupational therapy educators will be from COT accredited programmes. COT accreditors also assist the College in the quality monitoring of COT accredited programmes.

COT accreditors are appointed to the role usually for a period of three years. A COT accreditor should have at least three years' experience of occupational therapy pre-registration education. COT accreditors who retire or leave an occupational therapy education and/or practice role may be permitted to continue for up to one year after retirement. On completion of their term of office the individual will not be eligible to be an accreditor without a clear break of one year.

3.1 Key duties

- To represent the College at accreditation events held throughout the UK.
- To seek evidence, either through the documentation, via interviews or from undertaking visits to the HEI and practice placements, that the College's standards are being met.
- Make comment on pre-registration programme submission documents at undergraduate and postgraduate level in relation to the COT accreditation scheme.
- Identify areas of good practice in the programme as well as draw attention to issues of concern to the approval panel at an accreditation event.
- Provide constructive advice to the programme team, where appropriate, and assist in specific areas that require further development when accreditation is either withheld or not being recommended.
- Recommend the accreditation of pre-registration programmes that meet the College's standards through the COT officer to the Head of Education and Learning.
- Recommend withholding accreditation to a programme that does not meet the COT standards.
- Participate in review and approval/denial of minor/major changes.

NB If the higher education provider appoints a critical friend/external expert to work with the programme team in the programme's development and through its validation process, this person may not then act as a COT accreditor for that programme.

See Appendix 1 for a COT accreditor job description.

3.2 Criteria for inclusion in the COT accreditor register

During the process of recruitment and selection of COT accreditors, individuals will be asked to provide evidence against the following criteria:

1. Be a member of the BAOT in good standing.
2. Registration with the HCPC as an occupational therapist.

3a For clinical representatives:

- A minimum of five years' clinical experience.
- Active involvement in the education and training of occupational therapy students.
- Experience of supervision of occupational therapy students.

3b For academic representatives:

- A minimum of three years' higher education experience showing active involvement in the education and training of occupational therapy students.
- An understanding of current education policies and practice.
- A teaching qualification.
- A qualification appropriate to the level of awards being reviewed.

4. An interest in and/or experience of quality assurance of pre-registration education.
5. Experience of curriculum design and development.
6. Working knowledge of teaching and learning and assessment strategies.

3.3 Process for recruitment

COT will normally undertake a three-year recruitment cycle of COT accreditors:

- In Year 1, a group of accreditors will be recruited and will undertake training prior to the beginning of that academic year.
- During Years 1 to 3, accreditors will be offered roles as either Accreditor 1 or Accreditor 2 for a programme accreditation. Once an accreditor has performed one role they will then be offered an opportunity to undertake the other.
- Accreditor 1 will be required to attend an event, in addition to reviewing the documentation. Accreditor 2 will be required to undertake the review by documentation.
- COT will undertake, where practicable, to ensure that each accreditor has the opportunity to act as an accreditor in each of the three years. Every effort will be made to allow experience of each accreditor role.
- It must be noted, however, that conflicts of interest and accreditor availability can impact on this process.
- In order to ensure adequate availability of accreditors, COT will hold a reserve group, made up from the previous group of COT accreditors, who have agreed to act if difficulties arise.

Accreditors will not normally be appointed to more than two programme accreditation events per year.

Where a new occupational therapy pre-registration programme is being established or where two occupational therapy programmes are being considered at the same event, a COT accreditation panel will consist of two COT accreditors and a COT officer.

3.4 Training expectations

- Individuals appointed as a COT accreditor must attend a training day prior to undertaking any accreditation work.
- During their period of office the COT accreditor must read and engage with the annual accreditation update and the combined annual monitoring report.
- Following each accreditation the COT accreditor is involved in a quality assurance review of the event and will receive feedback on the process, event and outcome. It will be mandatory for the COT accreditor to engage with this in order to continue to act as an accreditor and develop skills and knowledge in accreditation.

3.5 Term of office

COT accreditors will:

- Assess and critically review course documentation submitted for the purposes of accreditation/re-accreditation against the College of Occupational Therapists' (2014) *Learning and development standards for pre-registration education.*
- Assess and critically review documentation submitted to the College detailing changes to a programme within the accredited period.
- Undertake accreditation visits to an HEI with a COT officer.
- With the COT officer, identify conditions, recommendations and commendations in relation to the accreditation submission and recommend the outcome of the submission to the COT's Head of Education and Learning.
- Act as a representative of the College and model professional behaviour at all times.
- Be required to disclose any known conflict of interest in the course of their work as a COT accreditor.
- Actively participate in the review and evaluation process of the accreditation scheme.
- Observe the COT accreditation processes and be familiar with the documentation that it uses for accreditation (a list of current documentation will be provided by COT at the start of the acreditors' terms of office).
- Be prepared to travel and be away from home for up to three days at any one time, depending on the nature of the accreditation visit.

COT accreditors act as representatives of the College and in doing so are required to model professional behaviour at all times. If an accreditor does not meet the training or period of office expectation or is deemed to have acted in an unprofessional manner, the College reserves to right to remove the individual from the COT accreditor register.

3.6 Remuneration

For one accreditation event, COT accreditor 1 will receive:

- 1 × day rate in payment for the review of documentation throughout the accreditation and for all discussion.
- One-off payment for attendance at the accreditation event.

- Travel and accommodation costs for attendance at the event.
- COT accreditor 2 will receive 1 × day rate in payment for the review of documentation throughout the accreditation and for all discussion.

For consideration of a major change, a one-off payment for the review of the documentation submitted and any discussion with the COT officer will be made.

For current rates please contact education@cot.co.uk.

Appendix 1: COT accreditor job description

A Purpose of role

- To review and assess pre-registration occupational therapy programmes delivered (or proposing to be delivered) by higher education providers using the College of Occupational Therapists' (2014) *Learning and development standards for pre-registration education.*
- To provide an accreditation outcome based on the assessment and review of pre-registration education occupational therapy programmes using the College of Occupational Therapists' (2014) *Learning and development standards for pre-registration education* as part of the College of Occupational Therapists' accreditation panel and to support the outcome to the Head of Education and Learning for final approval.
- To undertake accreditation visits to a HEI with a COT officer.
- To assess approved pre-registration occupational therapy programmes using the College of Occupational Therapists' (2014) *Learning and development standards for pre-registration education* during ongoing quality monitoring processes as required.

B Main duties and responsibilities

Duties include:

- Assess and critically review documentation submitted to the College for the purposes of accreditation/re-accreditation or ongoing accreditation against the College of Occupational Therapists' *Learning and development standards for pre-registration education.*
- Identify conditions, recommendations and commendations in collaboration with the COT accreditation panel in relation to the accreditation submission and recommend the outcome of the submission to the COT's Head of Education and Learning.
- Actively participate in the review and evaluation process of the accreditation scheme.
- Work collaboratively with the COT accreditation panel, the education provider and other relevant stakeholders.
- Undertake any other duties arising from visits or monitoring activities as directed by the Education Manager (Quality & Standards).

It is expected that registered accreditors will:

1. Attend and participate in the relevant training programmes for accreditors provided by the College.
2. Keep up to date with and apply relevant professional body policies.
3. Provide expert advice and contribute to discussions and decision making.

4. Commit to maintaining, developing and enhancing their professional knowledge, skills and competence through continuing professional development.
5. Conform to the requirements of the College's Code of Ethics and Professional Behaviour. When acting on behalf of the College, behave in a way that upholds the reputation of the College, maintain the highest standards of professional behaviour and be credible by stakeholders and BAOT.
6. Disclose any known conflict of interest in the course of their work as a COT accreditor.
7. Observe the COT accreditation processes and be familiar with the documentation that it uses for accreditation (a list of current documentation will be provided by COT at the start of the accreditors' terms of office).
8. Be prepared to travel and be away from home for up to three days at any one time, depending on the nature of the accreditation visit.
9. Endeavour to complete tasks in an efficient and time-sensitive manner.

C Person specification

	Essential	Desirable
Member of the BAOT	✗	
Registered Occupational Therapist	✗	
For clinical representatives:		
Five years' clinical experience	✗	
Involvement in the academic and practice education of occupational therapy students	✗	
Experience of supervising of occupational therapy students	✗	
For academic representatives:		
A minimum of three years' higher education experience working with occupational therapy students	✗	
An understanding of current education policies and practice	✗	
A teaching qualification	✗	
A qualification appropriate to the level of awards being reviewed	✗	
Other knowledge, skills and experience:		
Able to consider a wide range of issues in order to make informed and sound decisions	✗	
Understands the principles of quality assurance in higher education.	✗	
Understands teaching, learning and assessment strategies	✗	

	Essential	Desirable
Experience of being part of a PDT		✗
Experience of critically reviewing documentation against specific standards or requirements	✗	
Experience of working in a collaborative manner with external stakeholders		✗
Experience of attending and participating in formal meetings	✗	
Experience of attending and participating in large formal meetings with multiple stakeholders		✗
An understanding of current education policies and practice affecting delivery and development of professional training in a health and social care setting		✗
Able to explain and justify decisions and promote COT interests to all stakeholders concerned	✗	
Excellent oral and written communication skills and interpersonal skills	✗	